The Mindset Diet

Matt Rozier

DEDICATION

I would like to dedicate this book to all the people who have sought advice from fit pros and diet gurus, implemented it, and failed through no fault of their own.

It's not your fault that these 'influencers' were more interested in your money rather than actually looking to help you! You didn't fail, they failed you! I'm here to change that!

CONTENTS

ACKNOWLEDGMENTS

I'd like to thank all of the amazing people that have supported me in getting to this point! I've had some fantastic advice and support with writing, editing and publishing this book. Without your help this wouldn't have been possible so thank you!

I'd also like to thank all of the inspirational people that I have worked with over the years. Your journeys have helped me develop my knowledge and enhanced my passion to help as many people as I can, so thank you too!

Finally I'd like to thank the people close to me, you know who you are. Without your constant love and support I wouldn't have the strength and courage to put my ideas out there and chase the dream!

1
THE BEGINNING

Welcome to my first ever book, The Mindset Diet! Firstly, thank you for buying it (unless you have an illegal copy in which case thanks for the follow, but don't be so tight! 😊) I look forward to helping you make positive changes without giving up your life.

You'll notice that it's not a very long book and there's a simple reason for that, I don't have a very long attention span and I don't see the point in padding out lots of pages with info that you don't really need, I like to get to the point and then get on with it!

In this book I'm going to teach you how to unlock your motivation to achieve your goals.

There is plenty of information out there on how to train or what to eat, but nobody seems to tell you how to get and keep yourself motivated to go and achieve your goals. So, in the pages ahead we're going to look at what motivation is, what affects it and how you can put together a plan to maximise it for the best chances of achieving your goals. We will also look at why you react the way you do in certain situations and what you can do to stop it throwing you off course!

So a bit of background about me (spoiler alert… I didn't nearly die and you won't be getting a sob story, this isn't that sort of book and I'm not that sort of coach!), I was a happy fat child and I probably would've carried on that way if it wasn't for good old peer pressure/teasing/bullying. I was "big boned" as my mum would say at primary school, but not excessively fat so friends didn't really say anything.

It was only when I got to secondary school and there was a canteen that sold pizza/donuts/cakes etc and an ice cream van in the playground that things ramped up.

Also, there was nothing I loved more than going to see my Nan on a Sunday, having a coffee and dunking the best biscuits! She used to hide the good stuff for when I'd go and visit, she was the best!! With these advancements in eating understandably I put on more weight and before I knew it, I was pretty fat.

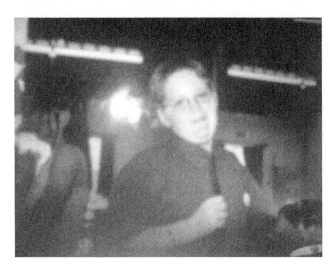

I found a love for rugby at secondary school and I started off as a prop (fat guy in the front row of the scrum), I fell in love with rugby on the basis that I was wanted because I was fat, brilliant!! Whilst that was great, teasing had started to creep in.

My name is Matthaeus {Matt-a-yus} which my family and friends shortened to Thaeus {tay-us}, and weirdly enough there was another lad in my year with the same name. I was a big fat lad, and he was little and skinny, we were quite good mates so often we'd hang around together. To stop confusion our friends decided I was "fat Thaeus" or, and here is the irony, FT for short because they were too lazy to say it all. *It's ok, you can laugh at the nickname!* So everyday there was multiple references to me being fat, which didn't really bother me in the beginning, but it developed into sound effects and then people I didn't like would join in and then I was bothered about it. This was over a couple of years, we were getting older and mates started to get girlfriends etc., then I was even more bothered and feeling left behind!

I realised that I needed to do something about it, and this is where it all started. I was about 14 and I realised I needed to sort out my eating and get my fat arse moving! This mind-set was actually really powerful and we'll look at it throughout the book. I wasn't particularly interested in health and fitness, but I was reasonably intelligent and could work out where the problem was with food, and it was obvious that I wasn't exercising enough. That's where it began! *Another spoiler alert, I didn't go on to win Mr Olympia and you won't find nearly naked pictures of me all over Instagram (I hope not anyway, they'll only be rugby related if there are any* 😁 *).*

I'm a pretty standard guy, in pretty average shape running a business and balancing life, whilst still playing, coaching and refereeing rugby.

Having said that, most of my big lifts (bench press, squat, deadlift etc.) are in excess of 100kg and I can do a 10k run in under an hour, and this is the basis that I like to measure my health and fitness. I want to be able to lift a reasonable weight, be fit enough to run a reasonable distance in a reasonable time and have a waist measurement that's a reasonable amount smaller than my chest and shoulder measurements! This is the attitude and mind-set that I want to help you obtain.

I won't lie to you, I'm upset (to put it politely) with the fitness industry, it's full of absolute shit! People are being misled left, right and centre, and that's just Personal Trainers and facility owners. You guys looking for help and guidance are even worse off. Don't get me wrong there are some fantastic coaches out there who can get you amazing results, but they are often overshadowed by show ponies who look fantastic on the surface, but they won't tell you exactly how they got to look like that because it will destroy their credibility! This applies to both men and women in the industry!

There are also so many fads, quick-fixes, 'experts' and 'opportunities' marketed relentlessly that seem "too good to miss" that it's no wonder you're lost! With no regulation in the fitness industry this lunacy and cowboy behaviour will continue, and it will grow. They are making money, fact! In some cases, quite impressive amounts of money, but it's at your expense and it ruins the reputation of the profession for the rest of us! That's what I'm here for, I'll tell it how it is, and we'll build a plan for us everyday people. If you truly want abs and a cover model physique (again we'll explore this later) then I'm probably not the coach for you, I've got coaches who can do it for you, but on the basis that I don't have visible abs I'm not going to preach to you about what you should be doing! If you want to drop a dress or trousers size however then keep reading, we can do that together no problem!

The bulk (no pun intended) of this book has been written at a strange period in life where most of the world is in lockdown hiding away from Covid-19. This presents many challenges for us in general, but especially for diet and exercise. There will be 2 outcomes for people when life returns to normal, person A will have remained as active as possible and been careful with their food/drink consumption and may actually emerge in better shape. Then there is person B who will eat/drink to cure boredom, buying in things that make them feel better, but will probably contribute to increasing body fat.

As you've bought this book, I'm going to assume that you are/have been person B, but that's fine because you are exactly the type of person that I'm here to help! So, on that basis, let's get started...

2
CURRENT STATE OF DIETING

The current world of fitness and nutrition is flooded with options and information. It's difficult to navigate the internet and social media without being faced with the latest celebrity fitness expert or hottest new diet. The world has become increasingly focused on body shape and various ways to get in shape and lose weight. That's not necessarily a bad thing, but as I alluded to in the previous chapter it has resulted in a lot of misinformation and poorly educated opinions in circulation.

As the market becomes increasingly crowded, trainers and coaches must do more to get noticed. Unfortunately, this has resulted in fit pros popularising methods of dieting that can be quite extreme, simply to get quick results for the purposes of before and after photos. Whilst participants do lose weight and fat in the short-term, these quick fixes are not educating and repairing relationships with food, often resulting in a rebound when people return to eating in the same way that they did previously.

The issue of education and repairing relationships with food is commonly left out of diets, and as I perhaps become more cynical in life I do begin to wonder if this is purely to bolster and maintain profit margins.

Let's look at the model of popular weight-loss clubs, I don't even need to mention names because I bet you can name them straight off! They have done a great job of creating brands and building a massive following around the world. They've also helped a huge amount of people to lose significant amounts of weight/fat and completely change their lives, and that is amazing. But what happens when you stop going to the club and following the programme? Often the weight/fat comes back again. Now I'm not saying that happens with everyone, and I recognise that most are probably still better off than they were in the first place, but my point is why does that happen?

Because rather than help people to learn about nutrition and learn how to manage eating, emotional reactions and changing habits they teach how to follow a system. They also demonise certain foods and attach negative connotations to ways of eating. This worsens the relationship with food and adds to the feeling of restriction, which in turn increases the chances of non-conformance.

What happens when you have something "naughty"? You feel guilty and feel like you've let yourself down. What comes next? "Oh well, I've already messed up today so I might as well have what I want and start again tomorrow, or Monday!" How many times have you said or done this?

For these reasons we must be smarter with restriction, and that's what this book is for. Restriction sounds like a horrible word, but in reality, that's what all diets are. They are dressed up and marketed in many different ways, let's look at some of the ways they do this...

Low-carb diets

Carbohydrates have been vilified by celebrities and trainers who often site them as the enemy for fat loss. The main reason for this is because typically most of us consume carb-heavy diets. A lot of the quick options we reach for are carb based, whether it's breakfast cereal, a sandwich in a shop, or a burger from a takeaway. They are often filling, tasty, and easy. This leads to them forming a large part of our daily calorie consumption. Therefore, if we restrict carbs in our diet, we naturally cut a lot of the calories we would normally consume, leading to weight/fat loss. The problem with this is that we also cut a lot of our energy intake, as our body prefers to use carbs to produce energy. So, if we cut carbs, we can feel sluggish and we may also experience strong cravings. We may also feel like we're missing out if we try to avoid foods that we normally enjoy. These two factors can be a dangerous combination when it comes to motivation. Add them together and they can be a real test of our willpower. Let's also remember that the outcome is simply a reduction in calories, so could there be an easier way to do this?

Intermittent fasting

This method simply cycles the body between periods of fasting and eating. So rather than restricting food types you just control the time frame you eat them instead. There are various time frames, but essentially, they are all leading to the same thing. Intermittent fasting usually leads to cutting out a meal from the day, often breakfast, so again it provides a way of reducing overall calorie consumption during the day. This can be a good method for people who don't want to closely monitor their calorie intake, assuming that they do not over-consume to make up for the lost meal.

However, restricting to certain time windows through the day could be unsuitable for those with busy and irregular days. For example, people who go from meeting to meeting throughout the day may not find a suitable opportunity to eat, therefore they may not be able to eat until after the designated eating window closes. So, before you decide to use this method you really need to consider if it fits into your lifestyle.

Meal replacements

This is the process of replacing meals with bars, shakes, smoothies etc. It is complete bollocks! I'm sorry to be so blunt, but I feel incredibly strongly about it. Yes, you will likely lose weight, and maybe even pretty quickly. But what does it teach you about eating? Absolutely nothing! How does it help you gain a better relationship with eating and portion sizes? It doesn't! Unless you're in a dangerous position where you have to drop weight quickly for a medical procedure you should steer well clear of using meal replacements!

Don't confuse protein shakes with meal replacements. Some people use protein shakes to supplement protein intake, and I've known people who struggle to eat in the morning to use protein as a way to consume calories until they feel ready to eat. In my view that is different.

What's the intended outcome of a meal replacement diet? You guessed it, to restrict calorie consumption. So, if you can do that still whilst eating enjoyable food why in the world would you choose a meal replacement!?

Paleo diet

This is sometimes also referred to as the caveman diet. It follows the principles of only eating foods that can be hunted, grown, or fished. It is a naturally high-protein, low-carb diet that eliminates processed food. It can be very effective for weight/fat loss and once you get into it you do actually feel great as a result of eating good, wholefoods. However, it can be a challenge, unless you are committed to food preparation. It's very difficult to follow the principles if you are eating out, or grabbing food on the go. So, you need to take this into consideration if this is your diet of choice.

This method is also slightly different as it isn't necessarily a calorie-controlled way of eating, that said you will likely still reduce your calories as you consume less carbs, less fat and less sugar.

If you can eat this way then it is a good option (in my opinion), but it is time consuming and it can be expensive.

So, whether it's restricting feeding times, counting calories, eliminating food groups etc, diets all share the same outcome, creating a calorie deficit. These methods have their fan groups, which also includes trainers and coaches who sell them, claiming all sorts of health benefits in an attempt to convince you that the method they are selling is superior to any other. But if you reverse engineer all diets, they still all share the same objective.

In reality it doesn't particularly matter what time you eat certain food groups, nor does it make a difference if you cram all of your eating into a specified time window. What matters is how many calories you consume versus how many calories you use in a day. If you consume more than you use, you'll gain weight, if you use more than you consume, you'll lose weight. So, on that basis why overcomplicate things with a list of rules and regulations!?

Food forms a big part of daily life and has a big impact

on our wellbeing. From social connections, to self-esteem and mood, food is a big part of who we are and what we do. Therefore, it is critical to our physical and mental health that we have a healthy relationship with eating. For this reason, we must be cautious when using restriction so that we can protect ourselves, whilst also setting ourselves up for the best chances of success.

It's time to ditch the systems, stop demonising foods, live without guilt and finally make progress with ease! Restriction doesn't have to equal torture! We're going to eat the foods we like, live a regular enjoyable life and still transform our bodies!

3
GOAL SETTING – WHAT DO YOU **REALLY** WANT TO ACHIEVE?

In this section we are going to drill down into what you REALLY want to achieve! "I want abs" I hear you say. Well, I want to look like Zac Efron, but 1) I don't have the hairline or the looks and 2) I'm not prepared to sacrifice my social life to put in the commitment that he does! That's the reality of it and that's what you must consider to create a SMART goal for yourself. There are a number of factors that you need to consider when setting a goal, and they will be critical to your success or failure.

1) What is your starting point? This is almost entirely centred on your composition (body fat %, muscle mass etc.) and you've really got to be honest with yourself. If you're currently 30st and 50% body fat is it realistic to set your initial goal to get a six pack? Absolutely not! Conversely if you're 10st and 10% body fat and you set a target to gain 5st of lean muscle in a year, that's equally unrealistic! Setting wild goals is the best way to kill your motivation based on the likelihood of failure! It's fine to have a big target in mind

as your overall goal, but you need to break it down into smaller targets to achieve along the way.

What are your lifestyle priorities? This is actually really important! If you go out for a drink every weekend, or go out for dinner 3-4 times a month, get regular takeaways etc. you've got to consider how important those things are to you! It's absolutely fine if you want to continue those things, BUT you have to factor it in when you set your goal! I won't get into Zac Efron shape because I like to eat out probably at least once a week (*in normal non-covid times*) and I like a drink after rugby, but I'm ok with that because for me I'd rather be social and in reasonable shape than antisocial and look incredible 😊. At the time of writing this (*when I first started in "normal times"*) I'm reconsidering my priorities and I've decided to only go out drinking once or twice a month because I've been out too much in the last few months, it's costing me a fortune, I'm a slug with a hangover and my body fat percentage is suffering 🙈! That said I'm not prepared to give up eating out because I enjoy it and I still want a social life! It's vital that you are honest with yourself and accountable for your choices. Your results shouldn't be a shock to you if you have planned properly and realistically.

How often can you commit to exercise? This is twofold - I'll use the word again, but what is REALISTIC for you? What exercise do you ENJOY and how often do you WANT to do it? I enjoy lifting weights and I'm happy to do it 3-4 times a week. I like walking and I can probably commit to that once or twice a week. In-season I play or referee rugby at least once a week so I'll be running on average 5km. Out of season I might play racketball or go for a run to make up for it. So that's roughly exercising 5 times per week. At this stage I'm not prepared to go to the gym twice a day. That's a realistic reflection on what I like and am happy to do. But you also have to factor in if it's possible to do it around work/family/social commitments. As a qualified

Personal Trainer, I'm supposed to nag you and tell you "there's always time for exercise" and realistically there is, but as a Mindset and Motivation Coach I'm telling you that if you're not up for it you won't do it, so it has to be relative to you and your life! Once you've considered both factors you know how often you can commit to exercise, you can then set your goal based on this information. It will ultimately determine the speed and extent to which you reach your target.

What exercise do you like doing? This is huge!! It's simple, if you don't like it then it isn't sustainable and you won't commit to it. It could work in the short-term for quick wins, but it's not part of your long-term plan so probably won't lead to you achieving your overall goal. If you like lifting weights then focus on a plan around that, if you prefer cardio do that, if you like group classes book in for some. Yes, there are some forms of exercise that are more effective or could achieve faster results, but at the end of the day this has to be something that you like doing so that when the time of day comes round to exercise you actually want to go and do it. You have to learn about yourself here too.

What's your knowledge like?

Do you understand gym plans and exercises?

Could you download a workout plan and go and do it without help?

If the answer is yes, you understand what the exercises are and you can do them safely then crack on! If you're a beginner and you don't have a clue, THAT'S FINE, nothing to be ashamed of, just get some help from a qualified trainer or someone experienced. Once you've got the knowledge and a plan the next question is

Can you do it by yourself?

Will you turn up 3-4 times a week?

If you've had a tough day will you still go?

This isn't a sales pitch, us PT's are expensive (if the trainer is cheap there's likely to be a reason for it, my education including exercise science degree and PT qualification cost in the region of £40k). If you can get there by yourself and commit to doing the workouts in your plan then that's awesome, keep it going and enjoy the results you've worked hard to achieve. If you're a "tomorrow" person and can easily talk yourself out of stuff then you need to suck it up and employ a trainer, or get yourself a committed training partner.

The absolute key to results is consistency, with the absolute minimum commitment being 12 weeks, but let's face it for most of us and our starting point (myself included) we're probably looking at a year to make the changes that we really want. I'm sorry if reading that has brought you to tears but this is a no BS book! 😊

It takes time to break habits and change routines and we have to factor in holidays and events where we say "f#*k it" and smash the BBQ and bar! I'm helping you to understand how to reprogramme your life, this isn't a 12-week low-carb transformation! But you have to understand it will still involve eating and drinking differently to what you're used to, because let's face it, what you've been doing has led you to buying this book, so you obviously realise that it has to change!

That said even though you're not on a diet there will still be times when you throw it all out the window and revert to type, it happens. Things happen that throw us off! The key is that you're in control! You enjoy it for the event, or even for a couple of days, and then you say "right, that was fun, but I want to get back to eating and exercising well now", and you will do that because the feeling of being fitter and healthier is far better than being slobby and unhappy! This mind-set is so powerful, you aren't walking around full of grief like someone has just died, you are in control of the fact that you relaxed for a bit, you made the decision knowing the consequences and you're ok with it.

Now you're making the decision to return to the plan you've made, you're in control of your results. With all this factored in we're looking at a year, maybe more depending on your starting point. But it's fine, Rome wasn't built in a day!! This whole book is coming from experience, sure there's some science and psychology in here, but this is mostly from the heart. The inner fat boy lives on strong and fights to escape every day, so I know what you're struggling with and the things I'm telling you to do are the things that I do, we're in this together!! ❤

Anyway, I rambled a lot there 🙊 although I hope it was useful! Back to training. There are so many different types of training

- ✓ Strength
- ✓ CrossFit
- ✓ Bodybuilding
- ✓ Powerlifting,
- ✓ Strongman
- ✓ Hiit
- ✓ Endurance
- ✓ Exercise to music and so on.

Those are just gym based, sport is also a major contributor to fitness and wellness. My point is if you tell me you don't like exercise, you're full of shit! Just the same as people who tell me they don't like fruit! You're telling me you've tried every type of sport and exercise and you don't like any of them!? If that IS the case then you're destined to be fat and unhealthy and it is actually your fault!

There is going to be a form of game or movement that you enjoy, I don't care if you're rubbish at it! I'm average at best at rugby, but I love it and I'll 'run' around a pitch for 80 minutes. It really is a case of the taking part that counts, the doing, no matter how good you are at it! If you're grossly overweight or terribly unfit it really doesn't matter! Who cares if you can only run for 20 seconds before walking again, or you bench press with 2kg dumbbells? What counts is that you do it, and you keep doing it week by week until it gets easier and you push to go further/lift heavier. You're in this competing against yourself, nobody else is competing against you!

I can prove this to you, I was working out by myself in a chain gym, on bench press, it was going well so I went for an extra rep, couldn't get it off of my chest 🙈 nobody even noticed, including people and trainers walking past!! I had to roll it down my body until I could sit up and lift it off! So yeah, people really aren't watching you as much as you think!

So, with all that in mind let's look at creating you a goal to work towards. We're going to use SMART goals. Specific, Measurable, Achievable, Relevant, and Time bound.

Specific - let's not beat around the bush here, what is the initial goal? Lose 1/2 stone? Shave 30 seconds off of your 5km personal best? Lift 105kg 1rep max on bench? (*I love bench press by the way, it's my favourite exercise and I make no apologies for using it in all of my examples!* 😄)

Measurable - how are you going to track it? Fitness

app? Workout diary? Pictures?

Achievable - Is it realistic? Have you set a goal to lose 3st in a month?

Relevant - is it in line with your goal? Does it make sense compared to what your overall goal is? For example, you want to increase your lean muscle mass, but you've signed up for an ironman triathlon. That's unrealistic because the volume of cardio training is going to burn some serious calories, and unless you can eat like an absolute machine and consume thousands of calories per day you will lose weight and muscle mass.

Time bound - set deadlines for when you want to achieve something by. This will help to keep you focused and accountable. But make sure it's realistic and achievable. You're not going to lose 10 inches from your waist in a month. But if 10 inches is your overall goal, then you can set yourself a monthly target of at least a one-inch loss. It's good to have an overall goal with lots of smaller achievable goals on the way. Success is a great way to build even more motivation, which builds momentum along the way. If you're achieving your goals and feeling good, you'll train harder, make better food choices, feel better and the results will get better and better!

SMART goals seem so corporate, but when you break it down it just makes sense to set out goals in this way. For a start it's just a great way to test if they are realistic or a dream! When you read it back to yourself do you think "yeah I can do that"? That's your test. If the answer is a true yes then you're onto a winner and you've taken a big sensible step forward!

With a realistic and considered goal in place the next step is to get your head in the right place too. It's all about your mind-set! To ensure you make progress you have to develop habits that align with your mind-set and your goals, forming these habits will be the difference between success and failure!

4
UNDERSTANDING MOTIVATION

It's simple right? The reason WHY someone does something or behaves in a particular way. Or the feeling of WANTING to do something, especially something that involves hard work and effort.

Those two definitions/statements really sum up the answer to successfully changing body shape. Firstly, you need to understand WHY you want to make the change in the first place, and then you need to determine how much you WANT to make the change. So, if it's that easy why do we struggle so much? We need to understand motivation a bit more so we can work out how to unlock it and use it to be successful.

There are several factors that affect motivation, environment can have a big impact and it can include physical and psychological environment. For example, walking through a shopping centre, there are food kiosks everywhere you look, everything smells and looks amazing, it's made even worse if you don't enjoy shopping as it will easily draw your attention. Even if you're not hungry you will be once you've looked at everything that is available. It's highly unlikely that you'll make it out of the centre without stopping at one of the food outlets, especially if you are with someone that doesn't share the same goals as you.

Which brings us on to psychological environment and your support network. Surrounding yourself with positive and understanding attitudes can have a big impact on your chances of success. If you are with someone who understands what you want to achieve and why you want to achieve it, they are far more likely to help you make positive choices, perhaps either through encouragement, or even by joining in with you, as opposed to that friend who tries to persuade you to 'relax' and tells you 'one little meal won't hurt you'.

Now I'm not telling you to cull your friends and family if you want to be successful, but we will revisit this point when we put together a plan to overcome these factors! Just take the point that environmental factors will challenge you and your motivation and you have to understand why and how you can prepare so that it doesn't derail you.

As you can imagine there are lots of theories as to what affects motivation, The Three Approaches to motivation include the Trait Centred View, the Situation Centred View and the Interactional View.

The Trait Centred View considers a person's personality and their individual characteristics as a factor for motivation levels. The theory suggests that motivation comes from within the individual, rather than from external sources. So, psychologists would agree that motivated behaviour is largely determined by the personality, needs, and goals of the person (Weinberg and Gould, 2007). In my opinion this alone does not determine someone's motivation, but it is important that you analyse yourself and you're honest about your own personality. What are your 'needs' if you are going to be successful? Do you need lots of 'little wins' to stay focused or are you motivated by bigger goals? This process will lead to lots of self-learning where you get closer to working out and understanding who you are and what you need to be successful. Wow we're getting deep...

The Situation Centred View is the idea that motivation is determined by the situation a person is in. This could be based on activity, place, or people, either contributing positively or negatively to how motivated you feel. For example, you may feel more motivated going to the gym with a group of friends to do a class led by a great instructor rather than going to an outdoor bootcamp in the freezing cold with a wannabe Army Physical Training Instructor! This is where you're going to have to learn about yourself again, you'll need to figure out which situation you're more likely to perform in if you're going to get results. It's natural that you will prioritise your time and energy into things you enjoy or you're best at, so if you sign-up to something that isn't really you then of course you'll end up finding excuses to avoid doing it! So, you need to engineer a situation that ticks your boxes in order to make progress.

The Interactional View considers both personality and situation together as strong predictors of performance and behaviour. It suggests that the individual's personality traits and the situation they operate in will lead to best performance. One size really doesn't fit all in fitness, so just because person A absolutely loves Zumba and has dropped 2 sizes since starting doesn't mean you're going to. You have to consider what type of person you are, what you enjoy doing, where do you enjoy doing it, how long you have, will it be with people, and if so who? I've left that broad as it applies to exercise and food, the same principles apply to both. Once you've worked these things out you can start to build your plan knowing that you've considered who you are, what you like and how you get the best out of yourself. With these winning factors you can start to get results!

I keep coming back to the idea of working out who you are, and what your needs are, it comes from two psychological principles: the motive of an individual to achieve success and the motive of an individual to avoid failure (Need achievement theory, McClelland, 1961; Atkinson, 1974). This theory is described as an approach-avoidance model because an individual will be motivated to either take part in (approach) or withdraw from (avoid) a situation, based on which feeling is stronger. If the chances of success are greater than the fear of failure a person will be motivated to take part in a situation. However, if the fear of failure exceeds the chances of success the individual is likely to avoid and withdraw from the situation. This is said to be a trait-centred approach as achievement motivation is a personality trait or relatively consistent way of behaving. Although this isn't likely to be the only factor affecting motivation, the situation is an important factor that could determine the probability of success and the incentive for success. People with low intrinsic (internal) motivation may be motivated by a situation with a high chance of success and a good reward.

Let's look at that in context… I've grown up playing rugby, I'm relatively confident but I wouldn't put myself out there as super confident. There have been many occasions when the testosterone levels have increased, and it provides a perfect example of motivation. We'll use arm wrestling as an example, I'm happy that I'm relatively strong, however I hate looking silly in a group, therefore my chances of success and my fear of failure are really battling each other in this situation. So, when I'm assessing which battle to accept, I'm weighing up how confident I feel against the person challenging me. If I feel I can beat the person (chances of success) and look good in front of my mates (high reward) I'm likely to accept the challenge. However, if I'm not confident I can win I'm likely to do whatever I can to avoid the situation. We do exactly the same when we select how we exercise, whether it's what class we join, if we attempt to lift a weight, or if we sign up for a running event etc.

On the flip side the theory also explains why 'high achievers' choose more difficult tasks as the value of success is much higher to them if they find it more challenging. Of course, this comes from a high confidence base which is why they perceive their chances of success to be higher and thrive on the added challenge. That said even if you don't consider yourself a 'high achiever' there will still be situations where you feel confident to take the more challenging option based on your skills and experience!

Stay with me here, I realise theories aren't exciting, but they will help us to understand why we make our choices and how we arrive at them.

To further understand ourselves and what can affect our motivation we have to look at Weiner's Attribution Theory (Weiner, 1985).

It focusses on how people explain their success or failure, given that most people look to understand why things happen as a result of the outcome. Attributions are generally categorised as stable or unstable (permanent or constantly changing) and internal or external (within or outside of our control). So, these factors combined mean that a success or a failure can be attributed to either ability or effort, or task difficulty or luck. The attributions we make are really important because they will indirectly affect our motivation by effecting our self-confidence and our expectations of future success. Attributions are generally either ego boosting (making ourselves feel better) or ego protecting (stopping ourselves from feeling bad) so reinforce our confidence levels to a given situation. This will affect motivation going forward as our levels of self-confidence often determine if we perform or avoid in a situation.

Putting it into a practical example I follow several people on social media who are members of a well-known weight loss brand, and each week they post whether they've lost weight, stayed the same or gained weight. Most of the time the post is accompanied by an explanation, do you see where I'm going with this? The killer post is when the individual has stayed the same and the post reads something like "absolutely gutted, I've eaten really well this week and exercised, and I haven't lost anything". We have to understand that we're working with an unstable factor here as weight fluctuates constantly, so despite the internal factor of effort being spot on, the outcome is largely external as there's a certain element of luck as to whether the scale reading will be different at the time of the weigh-in. You could even go back again the next morning and be lighter! In this case you have to understand that your perceived failure is not because of your effort levels, it's simply timing. Stay consistent and the results will follow.

On the flip side if you haven't made the effort (internal) then you can't simply blame luck (external) and use that as the reason, you have to be honest and analyse all the factors if you want to be successful. It's really important that you carefully analyse and consider your performance to avoid creating negative attributions that will affect your motivation going forward. Having learned about these factors hopefully you can now understand the statement "there's no point in me trying, I never lose weight anyway" and where it comes from.

It's also worth noting that when you're on a transformation programme staying the same is still progress! There will be weeks when the scales stay the same for the reasons listed above, but look at the bigger picture! You're still in a better position than when you started, as long as you haven't gained fat % you're still making progress!

Let's sum this up so we can put together our battle plan and understand what we need as individuals to make us motivated! I'm going to leave space for you to make notes (if you're listening on audiobook, grab some paper…). We'll make a plan for exercise and then for food.

Exercise

What type of exercise do you enjoy most? Cardio, Resistance, Martial Arts etc.

Environment

Where do you prefer to exercise? Home, Green Space, Gym etc.

Who do you prefer to exercise with? By yourself, in a group, with friends, with a PT.

Do you want/need competition from others or are you happy chasing your own targets?

Can you commit to working out by yourself or do you need an appointment with a PT/class/bootcamp/gym buddy?

Frequency/Duration

How many times per week can you realistically commit to exercise?

How long do you want to/can you commit to exercising? Is it consistent or do you want to vary the length of sessions in the week? Factor it into your plan.

Tracking

Do you want to track your exercise (time/weights/reps etc) or do you just want to enjoy a workout?

Food

What type of food do you enjoy most?

What food do you need to reduce? (Notice how I didn't say cut out, we're striving for a normal life, just not an excessive one!)

Environment

Can you trust yourself having these foods in your house or do the cupboards need to be carefully filled?

Do you need to take food with you, or can you trust yourself not to buy excessively?

Do you need to bulk prepare your meals or can you trust yourself to cook when you get home?

Do you want/need accountability from others or are you happy chasing your own targets?

Can you prepare your own eating plan, or do you need help from a professional?

Ok so we've got some answers, hopefully you've delved deep into your soul and you've been completely honest with your answers!! I do try not to be sarcastic; I'm told it's the lowest form of wit, but it keeps me entertained, and as I'm easily distracted it's necessary when writing a book!!

Although I make fun of this slightly, it is genuinely important that you've been truthful with yourself. This is your book, nobody else will see it unless you want them to, so take the opportunity to be really open about what you need. This is your chance in life to be completely selfish and self-indulgent! This book is all about you! Armed with this information we can create a powerful mind-set that will get you the results you're after!

5
A MINDSET FOR SUCCESS

Mind-set is absolutely everything for success, it seems obvious, but quite simply if your head isn't in it you won't achieve it! As I'm sure you know it's also really easy to be knocked off of your focus and then before you know it, you're back at square one wondering what the hell happened! The dangerous thing is that each time you fall off the wagon you negatively reinforce the idea that you won't achieve your goals and you'll find that self-doubt and low self-esteem grows inside. We have to act before you form the "what's the point in trying" mentality!

To turn this situation around we need to form some basic habits that will set you up each day and keep you on track. These are things you will need to practice again and again until they become ingrained and your mindset aligns with them instinctively. But once they're in there and you're living by them there's no reason why you won't be able to achieve what you want!

So how do we 'create a habit'? First let's understand what

a habit is. It can be defined as an action that is triggered automatically in response to contextual cues that have been associated with its performance (Neal, et al 2012). For example, automatically putting on clothes (action) after you get out of bed (contextual cue). Research is pretty consistent in finding that repetition of an action in a consistent context over time leads to the action being activated upon exposure to the cue. Or in other words after you've repeated a task over time you learn to complete the action when you're in the situation.

Once initiation of the action is 'transferred' to external cues, dependence on conscious attention or motivational processes is reduced (Lally, Wardle and Gardner, 2011). Put simply, once repetition has taught us to respond to the contextual cue, we no longer have to think about performing the action. We are taught when growing up to wash our hands after going to the toilet, after a period of time once we've consistently been helped to carry out the task, we learn to do it automatically after we've been to the toilet. We don't think 'oh I'd better wash my hands' we just do it.

Habit-formation advice is ultimately simple — repeat an action consistently in the same context. The habit formation attempt begins at the 'initiation phase', during which the new behaviour and the context in which it will be done are selected. Automaticity develops in the subsequent 'learning phase', during which the behaviour is repeated in the chosen context to strengthen the context-behaviour association (here a simple tick sheet for self-monitoring performance may help). Habit-formation culminates in the 'stability phase', at which the habit has formed, and its strength has plateaued, so that it persists over time with minimal effort or deliberation (Gardner, Lally and Wardle 2012).

Let's put that into practice. As I mentioned at the

beginning of the book, I'm writing during the lockdown period of the COVID-19 pandemic, I can only leave the house for essential shopping and 1 bout of exercise each day, therefore I decided to use it as a chance to sort out my hydration. I've been terrible in the past at not drinking enough water, one of my excuses is that I have to pee A LOT when I first start increasing my hydration and that isn't always possible when out on the road and busy. So, lockdown is absolutely perfect for increasing my water intake and training my body to get used to it. In order to be successful, I know that I'm very visual and I need to see progress and targets, so I got myself one of those bottles with times and levels printed on the side.

When I get up in the morning the first thing I do is go downstairs and make a coffee (I love proper coffee!!), but now I've added filling up the water bottle and drinking the first hours' worth of water into my routine before I have that coffee. So, I've got the action (having the drink), and I've got the contextual cue (first thing in the morning before my coffee) all I need to do now is be persistent and form the habit. But how long does it take to form a habit? "21 days" I hear you say, is that true or is it wishful thinking? Studies suggest that it varies massively from as little as 18 to as many as 254 days, but on average it takes 66 days to form a habit and change behaviour (Lally, Van Jaarsveld, Potts and Wardle, 2009).

21 days actually comes from a book published in 1960 by Dr Maxwell Maltz, and refers to plastic surgery and changing image. He didn't make it as a claim, he simply refers to the number as an observable metric. He writes "these, and many other commonly observed phenomena, tend to show that it requires a minimum of about 21 days for an old mental image to dissolve and a new one to gel." More than 30million copies of the book have been sold and 21 days has been widely accepted as fact, but it is actually a

myth!

There are variable factors that determine how long habits take to form which is why the timeline is so broad. It really depends on the complexity of the task and how quickly individuals adapt as to how long it takes people to form the habit.

Simple tasks, like drinking a glass of water before breakfast can quickly become habit as there is an easy action with a routine cue that is accessible. However, if the task is to go out for a run before breakfast, or do 50 sit-ups when you get out of bed these tasks are likely to take longer to become habitual as there are more factors that will affect behaviour change. The biggest factor being motivation! It's easy to go downstairs and have a glass of water, even if you don't fancy it you can still get it down without too much trouble, which is why it can quickly become routine. But going out for a run, or doing exercise requires much more effort and will require a lot more conscious thought and call to action before you do it instinctively!

That's why we're going to have to develop a mind-set that will provide you with the call to action so you can reinforce your motivation and succeed in building habits that will get you results! To do this we're going to look at some mind-set hacks.

Hack #1: Be clear on what your goal is!

We looked at goal setting back in Chapter 1 so by now you should've come up with a statement of what you REALLY want to achieve. You should've considered what is important to you, what you will change and as a result of that what you CAN and WANT to achieve. If you haven't done that yet revisit chapter 1 and then come back.

Write that statement here…

If your goal is weight/fat loss it is likely that your goal is actually a past version of yourself, a time when you were most happy. This is really powerful as a tool for motivation as it's far easier to picture your results when it is actually you that you want to look like! I found one of my old phones recently and took a look at some old progress pics I'd taken. It turns out that in 2012 I was in pretty reasonable shape, and I'm using that as my current target. I now have that picture on my current phone as a reference point so each month when I take my measurements and another pic, I can compare it to my target picture.

If your goal is to gain muscle/size make sure you've chosen a realistic example as someone you aspire to look like.

Either way be clear on what it is that you specifically want to achieve. A vision that is clear and focused makes it possible to achieve, if there are too many variables or you keep changing your mind you greatly reduce your chances of success, so take your time to work out exactly what you want. If it's a big drastic change then break it down into stages so you have a clear target to work to, and achieve, before moving onto the next stage. Rome wasn't built in a day, if you're serious about making a lifelong change then follow the process and be patient, it will be worth it to achieve that final outcome.

Keep the goal close to you, whether it's a picture of how you want to look, a picture of an item of clothing you want to look good in, a set of measurements you want to achieve, a bodyfat % figure, whatever it is keep it close. You need to see that goal every day, check-in with yourself and reflect on what your goal is and why you want to achieve it, what does it mean to you? You can come back to it any time you need a kick up the backside, a good reminder of why you're making the choices that you are.

Hack# 2: Generate a positive connection with your goal!

So, you know what your goal is, you know why you've set it, why you want to achieve it and what it would mean to you to achieve it. Now I want you to imagine what it would FEEL like once you've achieved it! How will you feel inside? What will that moment feel like when you look the way you really want to look? How will it feel each day you wake up and you're in the body that you've wanted to be in since you set your goal? Keep hold of that feeling! We're going to use it every time we're faced with a difficult choice. Each time you're tested, whether it's lacking enthusiasm to exercise or throwing your eating plan out of the window, I want you to stop, take a deep breath and think about what your goal is and how you'll feel once you've achieved your target. Then I want you to ask yourself if your choice is going to be worth it.

Be clear with yourself here, if you've been hitting the training hard and your body is telling you that you need a break then you should listen to it. Also missing the odd training session or over-indulging with food every once in a while is not the end of the world, the hack is really designed to stop you falling off the wagon and throwing your training/eating plan out of the window.

This is ultimately the test of whether you really do want to achieve your goal, if it really does mean something to you then this thought alone will get you to that workout or help you to say no to that cake.

We're working for a purpose here; we're taking control of our body and the way we think about eating and drinking so that we can be happy in our skin. It will also enhance the experience when you do have something you've been moderating from your lifestyle.

We know that when we can have something without having to make any effort to get it the satisfaction wares off after a while and it becomes less enjoyable or exciting. It's exactly the same with food and in particular sugar, the more we have the more blunted we become to the reward hormones released by the brain; therefore, we end up needing more to reach the same level of satisfaction. By being more selective with when we allow ourselves to have something, we will enjoy the experience of having it, making the most of the hormone release and the positive impact it has on mood and satisfaction. I have a perfect example of this which comes back to my love of going out for coffee. After I visited New Zealand and I was introduced to real coffee and cake (cheers Warren), I found myself having cake each time I went to a coffee shop after that. There is no excuse for it other than the fact that I enjoyed it, or at least I thought I did. Having it often also resulted in me having more and more sugary food, thus reducing the hormone response and also my enjoyment.

Also, in reality there is a clear difference between independent cake makers and mass-produced cake found in the chain coffee shops, if you reflect on your own experiences, I'm sure you'll agree. If you piece that together with the feelings of guilt for having it whilst 'trying to eat better' then it really wasn't/isn't worth it. This is where our mind-set and thought process comes in, I'm not going to tell you that every time you want cake you should think about your goal and how you feel and say no, instead I want you to ask yourself if what you're going to experience is worth it. So, for me if I go to an independent coffee shop and the cake is 'homemade' and looks incredible, I know I will make the most of that experience and really enjoy the flavour, so I'll have a piece and not feel guilty at all because I'm comfortable with my decision and think it's worth it. I can always play with my calories and reduce my intake elsewhere in the day to stay on track.

However, if I go to a chain with friends and I'm offered a cake I feel happy to say no because I know it won't taste as good as it looks so it's not worth it. I like to call this 'owning your choices', it's where you've considered all the information you need so you're confident that you're making the right choices. This way of thinking is key to making progress because it's guilt free thinking, you don't need to feel guilty because you're in control.

We've strayed slightly from the point but you've essentially got 2 hacks for the price of 1 there! Faced with any choice, you're going to connect with your goal, feel it, assess the situation and then decide whether it's worth it to you or not.

Hack# 3: Make a social commitment to your goal!

This is a good test of whether you're actually serious about your goal, are you willing to tell the world about it? You can't underestimate the power of social commitment, it adds pressure, anticipation and fear of failure into the mix. Now this can either work to motivate or intimidate you, and again we have to come back to your personality and what type of person you are. We've delved into that a reasonable amount so far so you should have an understanding of yourself and whether you'll thrive on this or freeze. It is of course up to you how public you make it, but you do need to share your goals with someone close to you at least, even if it's just the people you live with. Your fridge is a great place to make your public declaration, and no I don't mean sit in there and tell people every time they open the door!! Make yourself a progress sheet and stick it on the fridge, list your milestone targets leading up to the big one or set a monthly date to take your measurements and put it on there.

However you plan to track, put it on the fridge so it's visual to you every day and also those in your close support network will see it too. If you need accountability this is a great way to push yourself because even if people don't say anything to you, you know they will have seen it and they will notice if you've been progressing or not. More importantly you will see it, so when you can't be bothered all you need to do is look and see how much progress you've made and how you're getting closer to your goal.

Hack# 4: Own your choices!

When presented with any new choice/situation we instinctively react with emotion. It's likely to be excitement, fear or apathy. We either immediately say yes out of excitement before we even think about what/how we're going to do something, or we are faced with a challenge and instantly think of all the reasons why we either can't do it or can't be bothered to do it. After our initial instinctive reaction our rational part of our brain kicks in and reflects on previous experiences, as well as all the details to actually determine what/how we are going to do something.

We do exactly the same with food, we get excited and say yes without considering impact, or we say no because we don't fancy it (even if we should really have it).

So, with all of that in mind we now know that when we're presented with tasty food or choosing when, or if we're going to exercise, we should take a moment to let our instinctive reactions pass and then let our logic and rational thinking kick in before we answer. That might be after you've gone through some of the hacks that you've now learned.

Whatever the outcome is you need to OWN YOUR CHOICE! You can't afford to go down the road of feeling guilty if you have that piece of cake or resentment if you say no, you've got to be comfortable with the choices you make.

Consider why you're saying no, having gone through your decision-making process you've either decided that your goal is too important or that the experience isn't worth it. The most important thing here is that you've decided not to, you're not saying no because you "can't" have it, you're saying no because you don't want it. Conversely if you say yes, you don't need to feel bad about it because you're in control of the decision, again you've gone through your decision-making process and you can be comfortable that the experience will be worth it, and you can adjust things to compensate for it. I came across a great analogy from outspoken trainer James Smith, he describes calorie counting as having a daily budget. When you make a 'purchase' (eat/drink) you adjust your remaining budget to get through the rest of the day. I will add to this that when you get to the end of the day, you're either on budget (hitting your goal), under budget (calories to spare) or over budget, and in debt. So, based on these 3 outcomes you can set your budget for the next day around what you need to achieve after today.

This is the key to owning your choices and remaining in the right mind-set, you don't have to miss out on anything, and you can have whatever you want, you just need to make a decision on whether it's worth it and how you'll tweak things to compensate for it. For example, if you're daily target is to walk 10k steps, but you only manage 5k in a day, you could always aim for 15k the next day or an extra 1k over 5 days. By owning your choices and having a clear plan for how to incorporate them into your week and stay on track, you avoid the feeling of guilt. You won't feel like a failure, and you won't throw it all out of the window and go back to square one. It's a far healthier state of mind to be in, and can be the difference between steady progress and giving up again!

Hack# 5: Celebrate your wins!

Be sure to celebrate all of your wins, whether it's hitting a target or even completing a workout when you've really had to dig deep to go and get it done, they all count! Remember you're a step closer to achieving your goal and each step you make is progress compared to how you've been previously, so you deserve the pat on the back.

It's also really important that you take the opportunity to recognise your positive choices, especially if you have been tested whilst making it. Positive reinforcement can be very beneficial to motivation, and can lead to learned behaviour change. You will have seen this throughout life from parents praising you for learning something new, teachers rewarding your work with a good grade, through to promotions or bonuses at work. Rewarding effort or positive behaviour makes us feel good and makes us want to replicate it to achieve again. It's up to you how far you want to go with rewarding yourself, I would suggest that giving yourself some intrinsic praise and a metaphoric pat on the back is enough, but if you want to give yourself a fiver or treat yourself to an extra 15 mins in bed the next morning every time you make a positive choice then go for it! Whatever it is, just make sure you take a moment to reflect and recognise your win and give yourself some praise, this will help you to learn positive behaviour and it will make making those decisions easier!

Think about how you're going to celebrate when you hit targets, particularly which targets too. If you've set yourself a weekly weight loss target and it gets to tracking day, you jump on the scales and you've been successful it's probably not a great idea to celebrate by having a weekend long bender and eating what you want because you've hit your target! But it might be a good idea to reward yourself with something you want, or you'll enjoy, even better if it's something that isn't related to food or drink. We need to harness the positivity of success and use it as further motivation, not as a reason to relax and take your foot off the pedal.

As the achievements/milestones get bigger so should the rewards. Using weight/fat loss as the obvious example you could reward yourself with a shopping trip once you've hit your overall target. After all, if you're smaller than you were before you're likely to need new clothes! But it might be you treat yourself to something more than you'd normally have, maybe a brand or a style that you've been aiming for. Giving yourself the carrot of a reward alongside achieving the target itself just adds even more incentive to keep consistent and make progress. We're then covering intrinsic and extrinsic rewards to peak motivation! Think about what you'd like and put them into your plan.

6
MAKING YOUR PLAN

I alluded to the fact earlier that we initially think/react with emotion before our rational and logical parts of the brain can get involved, this can also affect our motivation. When we present our brain with a new target that is going to involve effort and perceived sacrifice our brain instantly reacts with negative thoughts! What it needs is a clear idea of how you're going to achieve this goal, what's involved, how are you going to do it and how long is it going to take?

This isn't the time for unknowns! So far, we've explored you a bit more and worked out the what's, the who's, and the how oftens (not sure that's a word, but it is now!) so in theory we've got the foundations for a plan, now we just need to build it up. Get that paper again if you're listening to the book, we're going to make your plan.

What exercise are you going to do?

What days are you going to do it?

Are you going to do it by yourself? With a friend? In a class? With a trainer?

Are you doing it for fun or are you going to track your workouts/sessions?

With this now in place, you can feel confident that you now know what you're going to physically do to reach your goals. Now let's do the same for your eating.

How many calories do you need each day?

You can get this figure from using a macronutrient calculator. There are some really handy websites that ask for your stats (height, weight, age) and then for your activity levels, and gives you the number of calories and macronutrients (carbs, protein and fat) you need per day.

Calories –

Remember to recalculate each time you lose weight, you need a calorie deficit to lose weight/fat, therefore, as you get lighter you will require less calories to continue progressing. Conversely if you're looking to gain muscle, you'll need more calories as your weight increases.

Protein –

Protein is the macro that you really want to hit. Not only does it help to repair and grow muscles that you've used for exercise, it also contributes to you feeling fuller for longer. So even if you're not weight training it plays an important part in helping you get leaner.

Carbs –

Carbs are always the villain in weight/fat loss. There is no doubt that if you reduce or cut out carbs from your diet then you will lose weight and fat, but that's because you're cutting out a lot of calories so therefore creating a deficit. But being a realist, it isn't sustainable to live a low-carb life AND be happy! Some of the best tasting foods in life are carbaliscious so why would you give them up? Carbs are also a primary source of energy used by the body, so we need them to perform in exercise and in life. In their simplistic form they break down to sugar so be aware of how much sugar is contained in the foods that you're eating. We looked at sugar consumption and how lots of it will result in a blunting effect on the reward hormone released. So, if you consistently over-consume sugary carbs, you'll crave even more to get the reward, which is likely to end up in overconsumption of calories!

Fat –

Don't be scared by fat, eating fat doesn't necessarily make you fat, consuming too many calories makes you fat. It's also used in cellular function and utilised by the body. So, if you're sticking within your target and not going over your calories have the full-fat version of whatever you want (except fizzy drinks!).

Are you going to bulk cook meals for the week or cook daily?

Do you need to plan whole days, or can you do it per meal on the day?

Do you need to take your own food, or can you trust yourself to buy food out?

Will you have similar meals each week or do you need lots of variety?

Can you create your own eating plan, or do you need help from a professional?

Can you cook or do you need to take lessons?

Actually a genuine point, do you know how to cook the food you want/need or are you used to processed food chucked in the oven? *If you fit into the latter mold, then learning to cook could be a game changer for you and your progress!*

So, we've got a framework now for how you're going to reach your goals with training and also for eating too. I would recommend the app MyFitnessPal for tracking your food because the barcode scanner and the food and drink library is really comprehensive and makes tracking so much easier. Make sure you set your own calories and adjust the macros to your goal as I find theirs is often higher.

Remember to adjust your calories and macros each time your weight changes. You don't have to track forever, but it is a good idea until you get used to the amounts of food and drink, you're consuming. I would also advise it whilst you're working towards a goal so you can be accountable to yourself and see what you did to be successful or what you need to change if you're not. Make sure you're completely honest with your tracking, you're the only one who will see it so if you really want to progress then you need accurate data to work with!

7
BUILDING MOMENTUM FOR MOTIVATION

It's really common to get excited (*I'm going to use that term loosely*) about getting in shape, once you've made the decision that you're going to start. You've suddenly built up the desire to take action, you set out how you're going to exercise, and you begin thinking about how you're going to change your eating.

Then you shoot out of the blocks with your healthy breakfast, you turn down the offer of cake at work and you go for a run when you get home, day one done! You repeat it all on day two, no problem. Bit more of a struggle on day three, but you get through it! Day four, breakfast was ok, but you forget to take lunch, you end up at the shop and you grab whatever is convenient. It has been a long day, you get home, and you think you should really get out for that run, but you're feeling sluggish from lunch and you just can't be bothered. You put it off until tomorrow. That's where you fall, your motivation desserts you and tomorrow doesn't happen either. Eat, sleep, repeat, and you're back at square one.

So, how do we stop this from happening? Question: why do you have to do both at the same time? If you're starting from scratch, then you've already got a big task ahead of you to either start exercising more or start eating better. So, why take on 2 massive challenges at once? Yes, eating well and exercising more go hand-in-hand to getting the results you're after, but that doesn't mean you have to start doing both at the same time.

How do you feel when you start something new and you begin to get success? It makes you feel good right? You enjoy the feeling of progress and you feel motivated to do more!

So, with this in mind when you have a list of things you need to do, or want to achieve, you need to be selective with where you start. Pick the thing that is going to give you lots of quick success. These little wins will boost your mood, give you confidence that you're making good progress, and you'll feel better about your chances of success. As a result of this you feel more motivated and ready to do more.

You can harness that energy and use it to kickstart the next phase. Let's take it back to the exercise example, and put it into context. Start by working out which one task gives you more satisfaction. Would you rather exercise more first, or change your eating first?

Remember you want to choose the one that you will experience success with the quickest. Use this energy to build momentum and then carry it into starting the other component. With your motivation firing, you'll then be ready to smash your goals on both fronts and hunt down those results!

By being targeted and smart with the way you start your

new way of living you really do set yourself up for the best chances of success. Not only will you physically make progress faster, but you'll also safeguard your motivation and protect yourself from falling off the wagon. It's a very simple idea, but it can be super effective!

8
PLANNING TO FAIL

Ok so now we're equipped with how you're going to achieve your goals, now we need to plan to fail. I know this sounds pretty crazy right!? But it's true! If you don't plan to fail then it will be a shock to you, and it could throw you off course, if you miss a target, or progress doesn't happen as quickly as you expected. Instead, I want you to have a plan so if something does go wrong and you don't hit a target, you'll know how to deal with it rather than letting it derail your mindset and your focus! Failure is an opportunity to grow, if you've made a plan and you've tracked what you've been doing then you've got all the data you need to learn from the setback and work out how to stop it happening again.

Let's use a weigh-in as an example, you set yourself a target to lose 1lb but when you get on the scale you've gained 1lb instead. This would be enough to throw Sandra from fat fighters into a spiraling mood blaming herself for not being good enough, and for being a failure. Or she'll blame the programme for letting her down and being rubbish. She'll then either punish herself by slashing calories, going hungry, and being miserable, or she'll go the other way and give up and eat anything and everything that she's been craving! But you don't need to do that because you've been smart, and you're prepared for setbacks. Armed with your data you can look back and see where you went over on your calories, or identify if you weren't active enough. You can then rethink your plan for the week ahead and adjust the variables, repeating the process at your next tracking point.

Using this process, you're always in control and you can easily deal with any setbacks you encounter because you're prepared for how you're going to deal with them. This is really important for your self-esteem and motivation, and you should adopt these principles to any tasks you take on. You've absolutely got to avoid punishing yourself! We looked at positive reinforcement earlier and how it can help to positively change behaviour, well B.F Skinner's work found similar results for negative reinforcement. If a child's first interaction with a dog results in the dog being snappy or even biting the child, then the child is likely to be scared to approach dogs in the future through fear of repetition. So, any motivation for being around dogs is lost.

If you believe you've tried hard in the week, but you've put weight on and punish yourself for it based on your feelings alone, it's likely that your motivation will decrease based on fear of failure again. So, we take 'feeling' out of the equation and just use the data we have! No punishment needed, just some minor adjustments and a plan for the week ahead!

We are currently living in a world where people of 'influence' to us (note that this isn't just Instagram celebrities, even friends or family that we admire count here) portray perfect lives and lots of success on social media. We only ever seem to see the glory and very rarely see any of the struggle that it took to get there. A progression graph is almost never a straight line, especially with weight/fat loss goals. Or in my example in the pic below, this is a screenshot from my Boditrax log at the gym showing muscle mass.

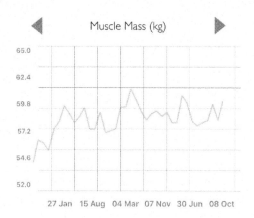

As you can see there are lots of gains and losses, all leading to progress in the bigger picture compared to the start, but lots of variance depending on how accurate and consistent I was with tracking, eating and training.

If you set out to lose 1lb a week for 12 weeks and you manage it every week then good on you, it's an impressive achievement! But if you don't, then don't worry about it, it's not a reflection on you, your ability or your effort. Life can, and probably will, get in the way at some stage; a birthday, a holiday, a surprisingly hot weekend that calls for a BBQ, why should you miss out!? If you're on a transformation plan, I'd encourage you to map out the time frame you have for your plan and include events like the ones I've mentioned. This will help you to factor them in so you can adjust calories/activity levels to work around it in advance, but if it's a last-minute thing you didn't see coming you can still work around it.

You've got strategies to get yourself back on track and the most important thing of all is you've got the mindset to stay in control and recognise that whilst it's a temporary setback it doesn't mean you can't still reach your goal. The great thing about having smaller goals leading to the big objective is not only the fact that they keep us accountable and give us motivation, but they also give us a real time picture of where we're at so we can plan ahead to see if we're on schedule.

The beauty of us not being Instagram famous, or booked for the cover of a magazine means that if we need another week, we can have it.

(If your body goal is for a holiday give yourself plenty of time!!! When I used to work on the gym floor, I had someone come to me 2 WEEKS before their holiday and ask me if I could get them results).

That said, this is only a contingency plan, realistically during a transformation you want these occasions to be absolutely minimal, you could get away with one maybe every 4-6 weeks, but if it's a weekly blowout I'm afraid you'll have to seriously add on time to reach that goal. It all comes back to being realistic with your goal, knowing yourself, knowing your lifestyle and knowing what you're prepared to change. If you're planning to go out and get drunk once a week every week you know you'll have to be pretty strict with yourself on the other 6 days to allow for it, and still get the results you want. If you go out say once a month then the things we've covered in this chapter will apply to you.

At the end of the day this is your book, your goals, your life, I'm arming you with the information so you can put together a plan that suits you and can work for you. All you have to do is be honest and realistic with yourself.

Anyway, that's enough about failure, it's a shitty word with shitty connotations, which is why I want to give you an alternative way of thinking about it!

9
TRACKING & SELF-IMAGE

Tracking and self-image are HUGE topics for me, I feel very strongly about both. They can have such a big impact on your mood and self-esteem, plus they have the power to make you obsessive with the results. I've lived with it; I've dealt with it with my clients and now I'm hopefully going to help you with it.

Firstly, let's talk about weight. Who really cares how much you weigh!? Do you walk around on a set of scales displaying your weight to everyone!? Once you've hit your goal is your best friend going to come you to you and say "oh my god, you look --kg" or are they going to say "wow you look great"!? The world has such an obsession with body weight and it's all you ever hear "oh I want to lose weight" but do you really? If I said to you right you can lose 10lb and not really look much different (*chances are you'd notice, but this is hypothetical so put your keyboards down warriors!! Lol*) or you can stay the same weight but drop a waist size which would you choose? What you're really looking for is shape change! You don't have to be a narcissist to enjoy people noticing that you've got results and point it out to you, it's a nice boost and if you work hard you deserve it!

For that reason I don't want you to set a number as a 'target weight' for your goal, because that number is meaningless. You do however need to know your weight as we use this to determine your calories. I do also encourage you to weigh yourself each week, BUT you only need to check if it has positively changed, not really by how much. Any progress is positive, but more than that, it lets you know that what you're doing is correct. Remember we are using this for accountability, and it also drives our data, we are not obsessing about the number because it doesn't really matter to us. When you're weighing in you need to be as consistent as possible, so try to weigh in at the same time of day in the same place, make sure it's on a hard surface.

I personally tend to weigh in after I've had my first bottle of water, I'm using bioelectrical impedance scales, so I want to make sure I've topped up my hydration to get a more realistic reading. Therefore, I make sure I'm consistent each week to get a truer picture of progress. This isn't the gold standard of measurement and isn't the most accurate, but it is accessible and gives me a good idea, plus it's for my own personal goal and I'm not aiming to compete on stage or appear on a magazine cover, so a rough idea is fine! With my readings I'm most interested in the body fat percentage as my transformation goal is based on that number. I'm not bothered about my weight, but I would like to be leaner as this will positively change my appearance.

I track this each week as well as my weight because it tells me what I need to know to adjust my eating through the week. If my weight has reduced then I know I've got the calories right, but if the body fat percentage hasn't decreased then I know I need to increase my protein intake throughout the next week to preserve and build muscle so I can get leaner.

So those are the weekly measurements I collect and track. Each month I will also collect measurements from my chest, arms, waist, lower belly and legs and put them into my progress tracker. I work out with weights with the intention of getting leaner, so I want to make sure that my chest and arms maintain, or grow, whilst reducing the fat around my belly and keeping my waist measurement down. We don't tend to see changes in measurements as quickly as we see fluctuations in weight, so I only do this once a month. I should have an idea from my body fat percentage how I'm doing with muscle, but the measurements provide me with feedback that I can take into my workouts. It may determine how I split my workouts up, for example it may determine if I do a particular body part more often etc.

I don't get too caught up with these numbers, it's just more data to reaffirm my plan or information to help me adjust it. I will then take monthly progress pictures, one front on and one from the side. Again, it's important to be consistent here, taking pictures in the same place in as similar light as possible. I use the pictures to compare as numbers don't really mean much until you can see the difference for yourself. But herein lies a potential big problem, body dysmorphia and self-esteem…

Body dysmorphia is classified as a mental health condition, it is where you spend a lot of time worrying about your appearance. By that definition you'd think almost every person in the world has it!! It goes further than that, often obsessing over a specific part of your body that you think needs improving and even viewing your body differently to how others see it.

Bodybuilders are typically at risk of developing traits of body dysmorphia, especially if they compete. As their body changes and improves they will move on to the next part that they think looks small, or fat, even if nobody else has

http://image.pollinations.ai/prompt/Matt%20Rozier

noticed it. It has also recently been termed 'Bigorexia' with documentaries and stories starting to cover the issue. This distorted view of your own body is what fuels the condition and can lead to eating disorders and further mental health conditions including depression.

These traits can also be present in people who have started a weight/fat loss transformation and have had some success. They too will look at themselves and see other areas that they think needs improvement. These people are at the highest risk of developing eating disorders to further calorie restrict in order to lose more weight.

As with any condition there are varying levels so not everyone who displays traits will go on to develop eating disorders and depression, it can be managed. This is one of the reasons why I use a combination of weekly weigh-ins, monthly measurements and monthly progress pictures to track my progress. If I can't see much of a difference in the pictures, I can back it up with the data of the measurements and the scales. This helps to satisfy my mind and stops me from obsessing over my body and planning how to either train more or eat less.

So, in case you hadn't worked it out I live with body dysmorphia, this is the absolute closest you'll get to a sob story from me! I'm not telling you because I want sympathy, the condition doesn't really bother me day-to-day anymore because I manage it with the data, I'm telling you so you've got a practical example of how it works.

I reckon for a period of over 10 years I said "this year I'm going to get a six pack for summer", and to be fair to myself one summer, when I was about 16/17, I think I got pretty close, before I self-sabotaged and panicked that I was getting too skinny and didn't have enough muscle. This turned out to be a constant cycle/struggle for me over many years, and to some extent is still with me! I've yo-yoed between trying to put on muscle, gaining some bodyfat and panicking about getting fat again, to losing weight to lose the fat I'd gained and then feeling like I was losing the muscle mass as well, and starting the cycle all over again! You can see a live example of this from the progress graph I used of my muscle mass earlier in this book!

It really does vary day-to-day as well, some days you'll look at yourself and feel like you're getting somewhere and other days you'll look and think "oh god that looks awful, I need to do x, y and z". This is why it's so important to have a clear plan that you understand and feel confident in. When you look at yourself and your emotional brain kicks in and panics, you can breathe and let your rational brain interrupt and remind yourself that you're working towards a plan that's going to get you the results that you want.

At this time of writing my bodyfat percentage is still a lot higher than I want. I was clearing through some things recently and found some old phones, looking through I was able to pinpoint the last time I would have considered myself to be in reasonably good shape, it was 2012!! Since then, it has been a constant cycle of putting on weight, muscle and fat and then losing it again, and then gaining it again and so on. The only trouble is each time I lost it I didn't lose as much as I had gained in the first place so my bodyfat percentage has been creeping up over the last 8 years. I think I was aware of it, but because I've gained a reasonable amount of muscle, I was sort of alright about it, and I actually think body dysmorphia can work in the opposite way as well. (*This is purely my own rhetoric, I haven't done any research into it, I'm simply writing as I think here.*) I looked at myself and thought "yeah ok, pretty good chest, arms and shoulders, could do with some work on the belly, but not too bad". General rule of thumb is if your chest sticks out more than your belly then you're doing alright...! But the truth is that this comfort zone allowed me to gain even more fat on my lower abs and around my obliques (commonly known as love handles) and this has only led me to an unhappy state.

Now I realise that I promote the message of being comfortable with yourself and I just said I was at a stage of feeling ok about myself so in theory there shouldn't be a problem. But you've also got to have a true picture of yourself and your habits and what impact that will have on your body. I know more than most what I should be doing and what impact my choices will have on my body. I find it pretty easy to gain weight, and fat, so I know that if my food choices contain lots of sugar and simple carbs then I will gain weight. I know that my level of muscle mass can fluctuate quite a bit too, so I need to consume enough protein to protect the mass that I have. In the period of time I just mentioned I was very relaxed with my eating and drinking because I had convinced myself that I was ok as I was and so I gained more and more fat until it was pointed out to me.

I am a rugby referee; I've been fortunate enough to referee around the world and at a fairly decent level here in the UK. It might seem like an odd thought to you, but there is actually quite a lot of pressure to look "good" when you get to a decent level, so when I started to gain fat around my belly and hips it was immediately pointed out to me. I am a training officer for a regional referee society, and we have monthly meetings. At these meetings various people will comment on whether I've gained size or lost it, and I don't think they have any idea what impact that has on me! But I have to say that over the last few months I've come to realise that they are completely right. To be completely open and honest with you I was able to literally grab a hand full of fat on my hips and lower belly and it was obvious from how my t-shirts were sitting on me. Yes, my chest and shoulders allowed for some weight gain, but the t-shirts were starting to hang differently with the lower belly and hips getting in the way!

So, after giving myself a reality check I set out to change it! I know this probably sounds like another cycle, but actually this time it is with a whole new mindset and outlook on what and how I'm achieving it, and it has actually formed the basis of this book!

I've been looking at how to create a healthy mental relationship with managing nutrition and exercise that looks after your wellbeing. By that I mean ways of thinking about how and what you're eating whilst avoiding becoming obsessed and on an emotional rollercoaster as you lose and gain weight. It is inevitable that your weight and fat levels will fluctuate, it's so difficult to be consistent all the time because there are natural changes in lifestyle depending on a whole range of things from occasions, to holidays, to life events that will throw you off or change your priorities. We have to accept the fact that there will be times when we'll be more focused and there will be other times when we relax.

So preparing our mind for this and understanding how we are in control, added to the knowledge that we can easily change things when we recognise we need to is so powerful and so important!

We aren't varying between the extremes of boom and bust, we're just raising and dipping above and below a steady maintenance line. When we're at the levels we want to be at we can relax our tracking and if we fall below our standards, we can pick it up again and get ourselves back to where we want to be. This doesn't mean drastic changes or "starting another diet" it just means being more conscious about what we're consuming again and realigning with how much we need to consume to be at the level we want to be at. This is now a lifestyle, it's freedom to live a comfortable life knowing that you're in control! It's understanding your body and what you need, what you can get away with and how you can change things to get the result that you want. Any time that you deviate from where you'd like to be you simply reapply the principles and hacks that we've covered through this book and you'll get right back to your target!

We also have to learn to enjoy the process, even in times of restriction when we're cutting calories you can still have the food that you enjoy! The only difference is that you'll make adjustments around it to accommodate a particular meal or drink. Learning to enjoy your food also improves your relationship with it in my opinion. I find that it also helps me to make decisions on whether I'm going to have it in the first place. If it doesn't live up to my expectations, I know that it's not worth the calories next time so I won't bother, but if I do enjoy it then I know that when I have it again, I'm going to really enjoy it and I can look forward to it and make the most of it.

I absolutely love a fruit scone with clotted cream and jam. I got some scones from the supermarket that were fresh and amazing, so I got some clotted cream and jam and factored it in to my calories for the day. I made a coffee and went to sit in the garden, the taste was unreal, so much flavour and every bit as good as I was hoping for, also really complimented the coffee so ticked all of my boxes. Sitting in the sun in my garden with some amazing food and good coffee is an experience that I love, so each time I have it I make sure that I literally immerse myself in the moment, eat slowly to make the most of the flavors and enjoy every bit of it. It makes it totally worth the calories!

To make it even better I understand how to map out my day with food/drink so even when I'm restricting my calories, I can still have these experiences. This is the breakthrough that I want to get across to you, restriction doesn't have to be painful, it doesn't have to be cutting out everything you love, it just has to be considered. You just need to be aware of what and how much you're having so you can work out what else you're having in the day to stay within your parameters.

Look how easy I got distracted talking about food...!! That said, it can have a positive effect on mood and wellbeing knowing that you're not living a restricted life, you can still have what you want without feeling bad. Having a positive and strong mid-set are vital ingredients to success, but also wellbeing! It's far too easy to become obsessive with results and how we look, so take time to step back, take a breath, look at how much progress you've made and choose to be happy about it.

Whenever you take pictures or measurements, I want you to focus on the positives first before you do anything else! Pick an area where you've made good progress and recognise the change and feel good about it. Then when you look at an area that you still want to improve it won't seem that bad because you're approaching it with a positive frame of mind based on progress you've already made, so it then just becomes the next area of focus.

I want you to add these tips to your memory bank, they are all really useful to building a powerful mindset that focusses on progress and success to continue to improve. We're about being positive and encouraging with ourselves, we're not about shaming and punishing ourselves, there's no place for that in our mindset. We're positive, powerful, progressive people and we WILL get the results that we want!

10
MAKING IT HAPPEN

If you've made it to this point then well done, you should now be in a far better position to get those results that you really want! This chapter is really a summary and a final bit of inspiration to release you into the wild to go and make it happen!

As you've gone through the book, I hope you've had plenty of opportunities to stop and reflect on who you are as a person, discovered what your needs are, what your preferences are and got an idea of what suits you best. I'll say it again that this knowledge is absolutely vital for you to make lifelong progress.

By now you should have lots of ideas about how you're going to exercise, when you're going to do it, who you're going to do it with (if anyone). You should also have ideas about how you're going to change your eating, remembering that you don't have to give up your favorite foods, you simply need to change how much, or maybe how often you're having them.

You should also have a clear idea of what your goal is too. Are you still trying to lose weight or is it really a body composition goal? Are you really bothered about that number on the scales or would you rather look and feel good? Remember to be specific with your goal so you have a clear plan of what you're going to achieve so you can add steps for how you're going to do it.

We know that our brain needs clarity and it needs to understand what the plan is to be satisfied and think rationally. (*Of course, I have simplified that statement, but it puts it into everyday understandable perspective.*) This will help you to think clearly when faced with difficult choices and will enable you to make choices easier and quicker. Note how I didn't say 'better choices', one of the biggest messages I want you to take from this book is about owning choices. To be successful and to protect your mental wellbeing we have to remove guilt from your food/exercise choices! Understanding what you're doing so that you can make informed choices and feel comfortable about it will transform your outlook and keep you on the path to success. Having the confidence that even if you overindulge or miss a workout you can easily adapt your plan going forward to cover yourself and stay on track!

The other big message I want you to take away is thinking of calories as a daily budget. This is another big factor to transforming your outlook and your relationship with food. It also makes the process far easier to understand! Knowing that you can budget your calories transforms the way you think about eating, especially for fat loss. There's no hiding from the fact that you need to reduce calories to lose fat, but working to a budget sounds so much more positive than being on a calorie restricted diet. It's also far easier to get your head around when balancing out a week's intake, particularly if you've had an over-indulgent day. If you've gone all out, had a take-away and a few drinks then it's likely that you've exceeded your budget and gone into 'debt', therefore, to get yourself 'back into the black' you simply adjust your budget for the next day, or the following few days to ensure that you recoup the extra calories that you used on that given day. Doing this enables you to be flexible with life whilst still hitting your targets and making progress. This is the secret to remaining in control and not feeling guilty and spiraling into an emotional mess.

Plus, we've also equipped you with 5 motivation hacks to help you make choices and continue to progress. They are...

Hack #1: Be clear on what your goal is!

Hack #2: Generate a positive connection with your goal!

Hack #3: Make a social commitment to your goal!

Hack #4: Own your choices!

Hack # 5: Celebrate your wins!

So, by now you should have asked yourself plenty of questions and you should have a list of answers. We've armed you with a goal, we've explored how you're going to achieve that goal and we've added 5 hacks to your toolkit to help you build motivation, gain momentum and keep progressing! All you need to do now is action your plan.

If you need help from a professional then NOW is the time to reach out, learn what you need to learn and plug those gaps. But make sure you start NOW, TODAY! Don't be one of those people that puts together a plan and then sits on it waiting for the 'right time' to start. NOW is the right time! Do AT LEAST one thing today, whether it's hiring a trainer, choosing a different meal or even just going out for an extra walk, whatever it is MAKE A START. Unleash that new positive, progressive mindset and set those wheels in motion. It doesn't matter how slowly you progress as long as you get started and continue to make progress.

Be sure to surround yourself with positivity too. This includes on social media, go through your feeds and unfollow any accounts that make you feel bad or share unrealistic images/content. Search for people that motivate you and share content that gives you value and makes you feel inspired to take action. Your social spaces should make you feel good whilst helping you to learn and grow as a person, you're in control of that so go ahead and freshen up your feed to match your new mindset.

All of these steps throughout the book will help you to create the headspace you need to fire up your motivation and move forward. Now is an exciting time for you so make the most of it and achieve the things that you've wanted for so long!

Thank you for reading my book and make sure you reach out to me on my social media channels to let me know how you're progressing and what difference your new mindset has made to you!

Best wishes

Matt x

SOCIAL MEDIA CHANNELS

Instagram: @mattrozier_motivationcoach

Facebook: @mattroziermotivationcoach

Twitter: @mattroziermotiv

REFERENCES

Scientific Papers

Atkinson, J.W. (1974) 'the mainstream of achievement-oriented activity' in Atkinson, J.W. And Raynor, J.O. (eds) motivation and achievement, New York, Halstead.

Mcclelland, D. (1961) The achieving society, New York, Free Press.

Mullins, L.J. (2002) managing people in organisations, Milton Keynes, The Open University.

Weiner, B. (1985) 'an attribution theory of achievement motivation and emotion', psychological review, vol.92, pp. 548-73.

Neal DT, Wood W, Labrecque JS, Lally P. How do habits guide behavior? Perceived and actual triggers of habits in daily life. j exp soc psychol. 2012;48:492–498. [google scholar]

Lally P, Wardle J, Gardner B, Psychol health med. 2011 aug; 16(4):484-9. [pubmed]

Phillippa Lally*, Cornelia H. M. Van Jaarsveld, Henry W. W. Potts and Jane Wardle, How are habits formed: modelling habit formation in the real world. European journal of social psychology eur. J. Soc. Psychol. 40, 998–1009 (2010)

REFERENCES

Books of influence

The Chimp Paradox by Prof Steve Peters

The Compound Effect by Darren Hardy

High Performance Habits by Brendon Burchard

ABOUT THE AUTHOR

Matt has been in the sport and fitness industry for 10 years working on the gym floor as a fitness instructor, and then as a Personal Trainer.

From there he opened a group fitness studio where he delivered classes and also went on to recruit and develop new instructors.

Alongside this he built a career training and mentoring coaches and match officials which he now does for England Rugby.

Matt is also a guest speaker, delivering workshops and seminars on health and fitness, as well as motivation.

You can find out more about what Matt offers at www.mattrozier.co.uk

Printed in Great Britain
by Amazon